Hypothyroidism Diet
[Second Edition]

Recipes for Hypothyroidism and Losing
Weight Fast

Arthur K. Burnett

Table of Contents

Introduction

What is Hypothyroidism?

Hypothyroidism is a condition which results when the thyroid gland is unable to produce enough thyroid hormone to properly regulate metabolism. Thyroid hormone is one of the most important hormones involved in the way that the human body uses energy from the food that we eat and as such, hypothyroidism has an effect on virtually every system and every organ in the body. An insufficient amount of thyroid hormone causes a slowdown in many bodily functions and it's a much more common condition than you might think — close to 5% of adolescents and adults in the United States suffer from this disorder.

There are many possible causes of the condition, including inflammation of the thyroid, genetic factors, damage to the thyroid gland from radiation treatment for cancer, Hashimoto's disease, a side effect of some prescription medications and too much or too little iodine in the diet. If you're afflicted with hypothyroidism yourself, you probably struggle with symptoms like weight gain, a lack of energy, dry skin, depression and sensitivity to cold.

However, there is hope for people who suffer from hypothyroidism. There are now several medications available which can be quite effective, although many people are becoming increasingly interested in doing what they can to manage the condition through diet and exercise.

There is still some debate about what foods people with underactive thyroid glands should or should not eat, although there is a general consensus that the best diet for people with hypothyroidism is a healthy, well balanced diet which provides the necessary vitamins, minerals and other nutrients.

What Happens If You Do Not Treat Hypothyroidism

What we do know is if hypothyroidism is diagnosed and treated early on the person will live a normal life, free from symptoms and ailments caused by having a "low" thyroid. Additional health issues are a big concern if hypothyroidism is not treated properly. For example, infants with hypothyroidism left untreated will not develop properly. They may incur brain damage and have learning disabilities too. Luckily, infants born in the USA are tested for hypothyroidism when they are born. Luckily, too, if hypothyroidism occurs after age three, brain function and intellect are not as affected.

If the thyroid is low from a condition called Hashimoto's thyroiditis then there is a chance the condition will improve and the thyroid will balance. Because this condition is mild, it may take a long time to realize even there is an issue with the thyroid. However, if the disease is not diagnosed and treated, eventually, the hypothyroidism will get worse and the symptoms of low thyroid will show up.

Another condition that can occur as a result of untreated hypothyroidism is called myxedema. Edema is swelling or retention of fluid in the tissues, so "myxedema" is swelling through an increase in fluid surround the lungs and heart. This causes a sluggish intellect (slow thinking) and sluggish muscle reflexes. A rare condition from myxedema is coma, which comes about as a result of an untreated low thyroid after years. Normally, this condition is seen in older adults who may not be having their thyroid checked often. The symptoms start with apathy and end up in confusion and finally psychosis. Coma occurs as the body temperature plummets and the heart rate slows considerably. Breathing is labored. It could also bring on heart failure.

Other complications that may occur due to an untreated hypothyroid are an increase in cardiovascular issues like stroke and coronary artery disease. This comes from elevated triglycerides and cholesterol that may be from the low thyroid. Adults may also experience dementia, fluid around the heart and even sleep apnea.

If the thyroid issue is mild, there may be no other symptoms for years. Still, if the thyroid issue is mild, it may be that diet can play a role in helping to balance it. Hypothyroid needs treatment with diet being a part of the treatment.

The Recipes

Since many nutritionists think that certain foods, especially cruciferous vegetables like broccoli and cauliflower may exacerbate thyroid conditions, we've left this family of vegetables largely out of the recipes in this cookbook. If you can't live without them, you might want to consider adding them in small amounts; many people with hypothyroidism can tolerate these vegetables in moderation.

The emphasis in this cookbook is on healthy, nutritionally balanced recipes which provide your body with nutrients which support endocrine health, particularly the thyroid gland. Almost as important is the fact that the recipes you'll see here include a lot of culinary variety. While people with hypothyroidism may have some special dietary concerns, it doesn't mean that your options are limited – in fact, your options are only limited by your imagination and your skill in the kitchen. However, if you use the recipes in this cookbook as a starting off point, you'll soon find yourself becoming an excellent cook and you'll be creating your own new favorites sooner than you might think. Feel free to experiment with these recipes and to adjust the amount of spices and other ingredients to match your own tastes.

As you would before you start any kind of new diet, speak to your physician to get their advice. Depending on the cause of your hypothyroidism and the severity of your case, your doctor may have recommendations for different foods that you should or should not eat or suggestions regarding nutritional supplementation to help manage your condition.

Once you have the blessing of your health care provider, feel free to dive into these recipes and discover just how much freedom you still have in the kitchen even as you keep your hypothyroidism under control by giving your endocrine system the nutritional support it needs.

One final note: although we've left out the word "organic" in these recipes, it's always advisable to use organic ingredients whenever possible. It's healthier in general and also recommended for hypothyroidism management.

Entrees

Grilled Pork (or lamb) Tenderloin, Puerto Rican Style

Number of Servings: 8

Ingredients:

2 lb. pork (or lamb) tenderloin, trimmed of fat
6 – 8 cloves garlic, minced or crushed in a garlic press
2 tbsp green onions, sliced into thin rounds
Juice of 8 – 10 limes
1/3 cup fresh cilantro, chopped
3 tsp dried oregano
3 tsp black pepper
1 tsp salt
2 – 3 tsp cumin
2 tsp olive oil (use extra virgin olive oil if possible)

Preparation:

Mix together the black pepper, salt, minced or crushed garlic, cumin, oregano and lime juice in a large baking dish. Add the pork (or lamb) tenderloin to the baking dish, turning to coat with the lime juice and spice mixture. Cover the baking dish and refrigerate. Marinate the pork (or lamb) for at least 30 minutes or for as long as 2 hours, turning occasionally.

Once you're finished marinating the pork (or lamb), remove it from the baking dish and discard any remaining marinade. Brush the pork (or lamb) with the olive oil and place on a grill rack (you may want to spray the rack with cooking spray to prevent sticking) and grill until a meat thermometer inserted at the thickest part of the tenderloin reads 160 degrees; this should take 25 to 30 minutes.

Allow the pork (or lamb) tenderloin to rest for five minutes, slice 1/4" thick and serve, sprinkled with sliced green onions and chopped cilantro.

Stuffed Winter Squash

Number of servings: 6 – 8, depending on the size of the squash and whether this recipe is prepared as a main course or as a side dish

Ingredients:

1 medium size winter squash (pumpkin or Hubbard work best, but any winter squash that you happen to have on hand will work fine for this recipe)
2 cups cooked brown rice (about 1 cup uncooked)
1 ½ cups dried cranberries
1 cup vegetable or chicken broth
1 cup pecans, chopped
2 tbsp fresh sage, chopped
1 tsp thyme
2 tbsp olive oil
2 tbsp ground flax seed (use flax seed meal or grind your own flax seeds)
2 tsp salt

Preparation:

Start by preheating your oven to 400 F. Cut off the top of the winter squash (this is easier with a pumpkin or a Hubbard squash) and remove the seeds. Mix together the remaining ingredients in a large mixing bowl, then stuff the winter squash with the mixture. Replace the top of your squash and brush the entire vegetable with a little olive oil. Bake the squash on a cookie sheet or baking dish for 1 hour or until it has become soft enough to easily pierce with a knife.

Remove the squash from the oven and allow it to rest for a few minutes, then remove the top, slice and serve as a main course or as a side dish.

Lentil Stew

Number of servings: 8 - 12

Ingredients:

1 lb. (one bag) dry brown lentils
2 cups vegetable or chicken broth
1 large yellow onion, diced
1 bunch Italian (flat leaf) parsley, chopped
4 medium to large carrots, diced
2 stalks celery, diced
6 cloves garlic, chopped
4 tbsp olive oil (preferably extra virgin olive oil)
Juice of 2 lemons, plus extra lemon wedges for serving
4 tsp thyme
2 tsp cumin
3 tsp salt
1 bay leaf

Preparation:

Place the lentils in a large stock pot with 10 cups of water along with the carrots, celery and bay leaf. Bring the pot to a boil before reducing the heat to a simmer. Cook, covered for 45 minutes. While the lentils cook, sauté the onions and garlic in olive oil over medium heat until browned, about 5 – 7 minutes. Add the sautéed garlic and onion, vegetable or chicken broth, lemon juice, thyme, cumin and salt to the lentils and simmer for another 15 minutes uncovered. Remove the soup from heat and stir in ¾ of the parsley. Season to taste with salt, black pepper and cumin and then serve topped with the remaining chopped parsley and lemon wedges on the side.

Poached Salmon With Parsley And Pumpkin Seed Sauce

Number of servings: 4

Ingredients:

For the sauce:

1 cup fresh Italian parsley, chopped (about 1 small bunch)
1/3 cup raw pumpkin seeds
2 cloves garlic
2 tsp olive oil (use extra virgin olive oil)
1 tbsp grated Romano or Parmesan cheese
Juice of 1 lemon
A pinch of salt

For the poached salmon:

1 ½ lb. salmon steak or filet
2 tbsp white wine (or stock) or cognac vinegar
1 bay leaf
2 tsp thyme
1 tsp salt
Black pepper, to taste

Preparation:

The sauce will taste best if you give it a little time for the flavors to blend together, so you may want to make it an hour or so ahead of time. Add the garlic, parsley, pumpkin seeds, olive oil and Romano or Parmesan to a food processor and blend until it forms a smooth sauce, adding a little water if necessary. Transfer the sauce to a bowl and add the salt and lemon juice, stirring to blend well.

Now you're ready to poach the salmon. Use a pot which is deep enough that you can immerse the salmon in it; fill the pot with enough water for this. Add the salt, white wine (or stock) or cognac vinegar, thyme and bay leaf to the pot and bring the mixture to a boil and then reduce to a simmer over medium-low heat, uncovered. The water should be just barely at a simmer.

Place the salmon in the pot and cook for about 7 minutes for each inch of thickness of the salmon steak or filet (measured at the thickest point). You'll be able to tell the salmon is cooked when the flesh turns completely opaque and will spring back if pressed. Remove from heat and pour 2/3 of the sauce on a serving platter, place the salmon on the sauce and top with the remaining 1/3 of the sauce and serve.

Peanut Shrimp

Number of servings: 2

Ingredients:

½ lb. shrimp, peeled and deveined
2 cloves garlic, minced
Juice of 2 lemons
2 tbsp olive oil (use extra virgin olive oil)
2 tbsp vegetable or chicken broth
¼ cup peanut sauce (your choice or make your own)
Salt and black pepper, to taste

Preparation:

Toss the shrimp with half of the lemon juice, a pinch of salt and a little black pepper while heating the vegetable or chicken broth in a skillet or sauté pan over medium heat. Once the broth begins to simmer, add the shrimp and cook for 2 minutes, stirring frequently.

Turn the shrimp over, add the garlic and continue cooking until the shrimp turn pink and opaque, about another 3 minutes (longer for larger shrimp). Remove from the shrimp from heat immediately once they're cooked through. Drizzle with olive oil, the other half of the lemon juice and the peanut sauce, toss to coat and serve.

Chicken And Chana Curry

Number of servings:8

Ingredients:

1 small whole chicken, cut into 15 – 20 pieces
3 cups cooked Chana dal* (canned cooked chickpeas may be substituted)
2 medium yellow onions, diced (about 2 cups)
6 cloves garlic, minced or crushed using a garlic press
1" long piece of fresh ginger, peeled and minced
1 tomato, diced
2 Thai chili peppers, minced (optional – you may omit this ingredient if you prefer a milder curry)
1 cup low fat yogurt
1 cup water or chicken broth
2 tbsp vegetable oil or ghee
1 tbsp cumin
1 tsp turmeric
1 tsp cayenne pepper
2 tsp garam masala, or to taste
1 tsp powdered coriander
2 bay leaves
1 cinnamon stick
A pinch of cardamom
A pinch of mustard seeds

salt, to taste
Chopped cilantro and lime wedges, for serving

Preparation:

In a large saucepan, heat the oil or ghee and mustard seeds, stirring occasionally until the mustard seeds begin to pop; and then add the onion, cinnamon stick, cardamom and bay leaf. Saute until the onion is golden brown. Add the remaining spices, ginger, half a cup of water or chicken broth and cook for another 5 minutes on medium-low heat, stirring occasionally.

Add the chicken, stir well, cover and cook for another 15 minutes, stirring every few minutes to prevent burning. Add the Chana dal or chickpeas and the remaining ½ cup of water or broth and cook for another 15 minutes, covered, stirring occasionally. Add the yogurt, diced tomato and Thai chilies (if using) and simmer uncovered for another 10 minutes, stirring regularly; if the curry seems too thick, add a little water or chicken broth and stir to mix. Once the chicken is cooked through, remove from heat and serve with brown rice, chopped cilantro and lime wedges.

Whole Wheat Linguini With Garlic, Tomato and Anchovy

Number of servings: 4

Ingredients:

½ package whole wheat linguini
3 large tomatoes, diced
4 cloves garlic, crushed or minced
1 tbsp olive oil (use extra virgin olive oil)
1 tbsp fresh basil, chopped
1 tbsp anchovy paste (you can use more or less to taste)
4 tsp grated Romano, pecorino or Parmesan cheese
Black pepper and crushed red pepper, to taste

Preparation:

Cook the whole wheat linguini as per the directions on the package, drain and set aside. In a large skillet or saucepan, sauté the crushed garlic in olive oil over medium heat for 2 minutes or until it becomes aromatic, stirring occasionally. Add the diced tomatoes and anchovy paste and cook for another 2 -3 minutes over medium heat, stirring constantly to prevent burning.

Add the cooked pasta to the garlic, tomato and anchovy

mixture and cook for 3 minutes, stirring regularly. Remove from heat and transfer to a large bowl for serving. Mix in the basil, black pepper and red pepper flakes, if using and serve, topping each plate with 1 tsp grated cheese.

Mushroom Crusted Sea Bass

Number of servings: 4

Ingredients:

4 sea bass filets, about 4 ounces each
2 tablespoons ground mixed dried mushrooms
1 tbsp olive oil

For the leek mixture:

4 leeks, trimmed and with the dark green parts removed
1 12 ounce package of crimini mushrooms, washed, stemmed and sliced thinly
1 tbsp olive oil
½ cup vegetable broth
Salt and black pepper, to taste

Preparation:

Trim the leeks, halve them lengthwise and wash them thoroughly under cold running water to remove any dirt or sand. Pat dry with a clean kitchen towel and slice the leeks thinly.

Add 1 tbsp olive oil to a large skillet over medium heat.

Once the oil is hot, add the sliced leeks and a sprinkle of salt and black pepper and sauté for 10 minutes, stirring occasionally and adding the vegetable broth a little at a time to keep the leeks moist as they cook.

After 10 minutes, add the sliced mushrooms and continue cooking for another 10 minutes until both the leeks and mushrooms are thoroughly softened, adding vegetable broth little by little as you go. Season the mixture to taste with salt and black pepper and cover tightly to keep warm while you cook the sea bass.

Grind the dried mushrooms until completely powdered; you can do this in a coffee grinder, a food processor or with a mortar and pestle. Sprinkle your sea bass filets with salt and black pepper, then coat with the mushroom powder.

Heat 1 tbsp olive oil in a large skillet over medium high heat. Add the sea bass filets and cook for 4 minutes on each side or until completely cooked through. Serve at once over the leek and mushroom mixture.

Curried Mussels

Number of servings: 4

Ingredients:

2 lbs. mussels, cleaned and debearded

1 medium white or yellow onion, diced

1 stalk (about 6" – 7") lemongrass, quartered and bruised

2 cups coconut milk

½ cup chicken or vegetable broth

1 tbsp fresh ginger, minced

2 tbsp chopped cilantro

2 tbsp curry powder

1 tbsp coconut oil

Salt and crushed red pepper, to taste

lime wedges, for serving

Preparation:

Heat the coconut oil in a large skillet. Once the oil is hot, add the onion and sauté until it turns translucent and starts to soften, about 3 minutes. Add the red pepper flakes, minced ginger and curry powder and cook for 1 minute, stirring regularly, until the mixture becomes aromatic.

Add the chicken or vegetable broth and simmer, uncovered until the mixture is reduced by about half, then add the coconut milk, lemongrass and a pinch of salt before bringing to a boil. Add the mussels and lower the heat to medium. Cover and cook for 7 minutes, then check for doneness – remove and discard any mussels which are still closed at this point. Serve in individual bowls with the curry broth and topped with chopped cilantro and lime wedges on the side.

Turkey Burgers

Number of servings: 4

Ingredients:

1 lb. ground turkey

¼ of a small white onion, minced

1 slice whole grain bread, toasted

2 cloves garlic, minced

1 tbsp fresh Italian parsley, minced

½ tsp basil

½ tsp oregano

½ tsp black pepper

½ tsp salt

1 egg white

Preparation:

Start by making breadcrumbs. Toast the slice of whole grain bread and add to a food processor along with the oregano and basil. Grind into coarse crumbs and transfer to a large bowl along with the minced onion, egg white, minced parsley, minced garlic, ground turkey, salt and black pepper. Mix together well and form into patties – you should have enough of the mixture to make 4 turkey burger patties.

In a nonstick skillet, cook the patties until they measure 180 F in the center when tested with a meat thermometer. Serve on whole grain buns with the toppings and condiments of your choice.

Eggplant Rolls

Number of servings: 4

Ingredients:

1 large eggplant

2 cups arugula, chopped

1 cup fresh basil, chopped

1 cup ricotta cheese

1 cup (8 ounces) cream cheese, softened at room temperature

3 cloves garlic, minced

6 sun dried tomatoes, chopped finely

4 ounces Parmesan or Romano cheese, grated

Black pepper, to taste

Preparation:

Heat a grill (either an outdoor charcoal grill or a grill pan on the stove) while you slice the eggplant very thinly and sprinkle each slice with a pinch of salt. If you're grilling the eggplant on a charcoal grill, brush them with a little olive oil to keep them from sticking to the grill while they cook. Grill each slice for about 2 minutes per side until just cooked through.

Once the eggplant slices are cooked, mix together the softened cream cheese, ricotta cheese, chopped sun dried tomatoes, minced garlic and a generous amount of black pepper. Top each slice of grilled eggplant with about spoonful of the cheese mixture and some of the chopped basil and arugula. Roll up each filled eggplant slice into a roll and serve.

Chicken With Mushrooms in Sauce

Ingredients:

4 chicken legs

4 shallots, minced

1 cup sliced crimini or button mushrooms

4 cloves garlic, minced

2 cups chicken broth

1 cup dry red wine (or stock)

2 tbsp butter

1 tbsp tomato paste

1 tbsp olive oil

2 tsp marjoram

1 tsp oregano

Salt and black pepper, to taste

Preparation:

Using kitchen shears, separate the chicken into thighs and drumsticks. Pat the chicken dry with paper towels and season with a little salt and black pepper. Melt the butter over medium heat in a large stock pot or Dutch oven and brown the chicken (you'll probably need to do this in batches); remove the chicken when it's browned and set aside.

Add the minced shallots and garlic to the pot and sauté for about 5 minutes or until softened and translucent. Add the tomato paste and continue cooking for 1 minute, then add the wine (or stock) and turn up the heat to high. Bring to a boil and cook until the wine (or stock) is reduced by about half; this will take 3 – 5 minutes.

Once the wine (or stock) is reduced by half, add the mushrooms, chicken and chicken broth and reduce the heat to low and simmer, partially covered, until the chicken is cooked and the sauce has thickened. Stir in the marjoram and oregano and season to taste with salt and black pepper before serving.

Rouladen

Number of servings: 6

Ingredients:

1 ½ lbs. flank steak
6 slices bacon (applewood smoked bacon is especially good for this recipe)
2 ½ cups beef stock
2 medium red onions, sliced thinly
4 dill pickle spears, sliced thinly
8 tsp brown mustard
2 tbsp butter

Preparation:

Note: You'll need a very sharp knife for this recipe, both to cut the steak and to slice the pickles and onions as thinly as possible.

Slice the flank steak into 6 slices about 3" wide and ¼" thick. Slice the pickles thinly lengthwise. Peel the onions, halve them and slice very thinly.

Next, lay out the strips of flank steak on a cutting board or other clean work surface and spread each strip with about 1 tsp of brown mustard (or more, if desired). Top each strip with a slice of bacon, followed by slices of onion and pickle. Roll the slices up tightly and pin them together with a toothpick.

Melt the butter in a cast iron skillet over medium heat. Cook the rolls for 2 minutes on each side to brown them. Once the roulades are browned, add the beef broth, reduce the heat to a simmer and cover. Simmer for one hour, covered. Allow the roulades to rest for a few minutes and serve.

Clams Oreganata

Number of servings: 4

Ingredients:

2 lbs. small clams, well-scrubbed and rinsed

¼ cup vegetable or chicken broth

4 Roma tomatoes, diced

4 cloves garlic, minced

2 tbsp fresh oregano, chopped

Zest of 1 lemon

1 slice of whole grain bread

Lemon wedges, for serving

Preparation:

The first step is to make breadcrumbs. Toast the slice of wholegrain bread and grind into crumbs in a food processor along with the lemon zest and 1 tbsp of oregano.

Add the vegetable or chicken broth and garlic to a large saucepan or stockpot and heat over medium low heat until the garlic becomes aromatic, about 2 minutes. Add the tomatoes and the remaining 1 tbsp or oregano and cook, stirring regularly for about 5 minutes until the tomatoes soften and start to break down.

Add the clams and stir well. Add another splash of broth, cover the pot and turn up the heat to medium and cook for 7 minutes. Remove and discard any clams which have not opened after being cooked for 7 minutes.

Divide the clams and the remaining broth into soup bowls and serve, sprinkled with the bread crumb mixture.

Horseradish-Almond Crusted Salmon

Number of servings: 6

Ingredients:

6 salmon filets, about 6 ounces each
8 tbsp horseradish
1 shallot, minced
1 tbsp extra virgin olive oil
½ cup almond flour
2 tbsp chopped dill
1 tsp salt
Black pepper, to taste

Preparation:

Start by preheating your oven to 450 F. In a medium sized bowl, mix together the almond flour, ½ tsp salt, a generous sprinkle of black pepper, the minced shallot, chopped dill, olive oil and the horseradish. Mix well to combine the ingredients and set the mixture aside.

Lightly oil a large baking pan with olive oil or cooking spray and place the salmon filets on the pan, making sure that the filets do not touch each other. Season the salmon filets with the other ½ tsp salt and plenty of black pepper. Spread each salmon filet with the horseradish mixture and bake for 5 minutes or until the salmon is just cooked through. Turn the oven to a broil and cook until the tops are nicely browned, about 2 minutes. Remove from the oven and serve immediately.

Roast Pork (or lamb) With Fennel

Number of servings: 8

Ingredients:

2 lbs. pork (or lamb) loin
8 cloves garlic, crushed
1/3 cup fresh rosemary
1 tbsp Dijon mustard
2 tbsp lemon zest
2 tbsp olive oil
2 tsp fennel seeds
Salt and black pepper, to taste

Preparation:

Start by preheating your oven to 400 F. Put the pork (or lamb) loin in a baking dish, fatty side facing up. Grind the garlic, rosemary, lemon zest and fennel coarsely in a food processor, then add the mustard, olive oil and a little salt and pepper to the mixture and continue processing until it forms a smooth paste. Brush the mustard, garlic and herb mixture on the pork (or lamb) loin.

Place the pork (or lamb) loin in the oven and cook for 1

hour or until a meat thermometer inserted at the thickest part reads at least 140 F. Remove the pork (or lamb) loin from the oven and let it rest for 20 minutes before slicing and serving.

Spaghetti Squash With Buffalo Bolognese

Ingredients:

1 medium sized spaghetti squash
1 lb. ground buffalo
1 green bell pepper, diced
1 large yellow onion, diced
4 large tomatoes, diced
4 cloves garlic, minced
2 tsp oregano
2 tsp olive oil
Salt and black pepper, to taste

Preparation:

Preheat your oven to 400 F. Pierce the spaghetti squash in a few places and once the oven has reached 400 F, place the squash on a baking sheet and bake for 1 hour.

While the spaghetti squash is baking, heat the olive oil in

a large skillet over high heat. Once the skillet is hot, add the ground buffalo and cook for 5 minutes, stirring occasionally. Drain off the fat and discard, then add in the diced tomatoes, diced green pepper, minced garlic, oregano and a little black pepper. Bring the mixture to a boil and then reduce to medium low and simmer, covered, stirring occasionally. Cook for another 15 minutes uncovered, stirring regularly.

Once the spaghetti squash is done, remove from the oven, cut in half lengthwise and allow to cool for a few minutes. Scoop out the seeds and separate the flesh into strands using a fork. Place a portion of the spaghetti squash on individual plates, top with the buffalo sauce and serve.

Stuffed Poblano Peppers With Crab, Goat Cheese And Mango Salsa

Number of servings: 8

Ingredients:

8 poblano peppers

1 6 ounce can crabmeat, drained and rinsed (jumbo lump crabmeat is best)

8 ounces Oaxaca or mozzarella cheese, shredded

4 ounces goat cheese

1 cup corn (frozen and thawed or home cooked and cut from the cob)

1 small yellow onion, minced

2 cloves garlic, minced

2 egg whites (from large or extra-large eggs)

1 tsp cumin

2 tbsp olive oil

Black pepper, to taste

For the mango salsa:

2 mangoes, peeled, seeded and diced

1/3 cup fresh cilantro, chopped

½ of a small red onion, minced

Juice of 2 -3 limes

2 tbsp orange juice

A dash of olive oil

Preparation:

Start by making the mango salsa. Mix together the diced mango, minced red onion, olive oil, lime juice and orange juice in a plastic or ceramic bowl (metal bowls may react with the acid in the citrus juices and give your salsa an unpleasant metallic taste). Refrigerate for at least 2 hours to allow the flavors to combine.

Next, heat your oven to broiling temperature. Line a baking dish or cookie sheet with aluminum foil and broil the poblano peppers for 5 minutes per side or until they blister. Remove the poblanos from the oven and place in a large paper bag; close the bag tightly and allow them to steam in the bag for 10 minutes to loosen their skins. Place the peppers under cold running water, rubbing them gently – the skins should slip off easily.

Slice the peppers open lengthwise on one side, keeping the stems in place. Remove the seeds and pith from the peppers and discard, then set the poblano peppers aside to cool.

Heat your oven to 375 F while you prepare the crabmeat filling. Beat the egg whites in a bowl until frothy, then place in a food processor along with the goat cheese, Oaxaca or mozzarella cheese, cumin and black pepper and process until blended. Transfer the cheese mixture to a bowl and mix in the corn and drained crabmeat.

Divide the crabmeat and cheese mixture evenly among the peppers and pinch the edges of the peppers together to seal; you can also use toothpicks to close the cut edges if necessary.

Place the stuffed poblanos in a large baking dish coated with olive oil or cooking spray with the seam sides down. Cover the dish with aluminum foil and bake for 30 minutes. Serve the stuffed peppers with mango salsa and serve.

Stuffed Zucchini With Shrimp And Feta Cheese

Number of servings: 6

Ingredients:

6 small to medium zucchini or yellow squash, cut in half lengthwise
¾ lb. shrimp, peeled and deveined
1 medium tomato, diced
1 medium red bell pepper, diced finely
2 cloves garlic, minced
1 small red onion, diced finely
2/3 cup (about 6 ounces) feta cheese, crumbled
2 tbsp fresh Italian parsley, chopped
2 tbsp fresh dill, chopped
2 tbsp olive oil (use extra virgin olive oil)
Salt, black pepper and crushed red pepper, to taste

Preparation:

Preheat your oven to 425 F. While the oven heats, fill a medium pot about halfway with water and bring to a boil. Boil the shrimp for about 5 minutes or until it's cooked through (it will be opaque once it's cooked). Remove from heat, drain and chop the shrimp finely.

Heat the olive oil in a skillet over medium high heat and sauté the onion, garlic and red bell pepper until tender, about 5 minutes. Add the diced tomatoes and a little crushed red pepper, if using and cook over medium heat until the mixture thickens, about 5 minutes, stirring regularly. Remove from heat and season to taste with salt and black pepper, then stir in the chopped shrimp, dill and parsley.

Scoop out most of the flesh from the zucchini or yellow squash halves, leaving about ¼" behind. Rub the squash halves with olive oil, stuff with the tomato and shrimp mixture, then top with crumbled feta cheese.

Place the stuffed zucchini on a lightly oiled baking sheet and cook for 30 minutes, until the zucchini starts to become tender and the feta cheese is lightly browned, remove from the oven and serve hot.

Fish Tacos

Ingredients:

1 lb. halibut
4 tbsp taco sauce (any kind you like)
1 small white onion, diced
½ cup shredded cheese (optional)
½ cup sour cream (optional)
4 tortillas
Salsa and lime wedges, for serving

Preparation:

Heat your oven to broiling temperature. While the oven is heating, brush the halibut with the taco sauce and place on a baking sheet. Broil for 5 minutes, then turn over and broil for another 5 minutes or until the fish turns completely opaque and flakes easily with a fork.

Remove the halibut from the oven and transfer to a bowl. Flake the fish with a fork and set aside. Toast the tortillas over the flame of a gas stove; you can also heat them on a dry skillet for a few seconds per side over high heat or warm them in the microwave if you don't have a gas stove.

Divide the flaked halibut among the tortillas and top with diced onion, salsa, cheese and sour cream (if using) squeeze a lime wedge over each taco and serve.

Chicken Puttanesca

Number of servings: 4

Ingredients:

4 chicken breasts, about 4 ounces each
2 tomatoes, diced
6 cloves garlic, minced
½ cup kalamata olives, chopped
2 tbsp fresh basil, chopped
2 tbsp capers
Juice of 1 lemon
4 tsp olive oil
Salt, black pepper and red pepper flakes, to taste

Preparation:

Set your oven to warm. Heat 2 tsp olive oil in a large skillet over medium high heat; while the oil heats, season the chicken breasts with salt and pepper. Cook the chicken breasts for 2 minutes or until browned, turn over and cook for another 30 seconds. Remove the chicken breasts from the pan and transfer to a baking dish and place in the oven to keep warm.

Add the other 2 tsp of olive oil to the skillet and sauté

the garlic over medium heat for 1 minute or until it becomes aromatic, stirring regularly. Add the diced tomatoes, chopped olives, capers and pepper flakes to taste and simmer for 5 minutes until the sauce thickens slightly. Stir regularly to break up the tomatoes as they cook. Stir in the basil and lemon juice and remove from heat. Season to taste with salt, black pepper and crushed red pepper.

Take the chicken breasts out of the oven and transfer to individual plates. Top each chicken breast with a portion of the puttanesca sauce and serve.

Brandied Beef Tenderloin

Number of servings: 4

Ingredients:

4 beef tenderloin filets (about 4 ounces each)
½ cup beef stock
3 tbsp fresh Italian parsley, chopped
3 cloves garlic, minced
½ tbsp butter
1 tbsp olive oil
2 ounces brandy or cognac
Salt and black pepper, to taste

Preparation:

Season the beef tenderloin filets with salt and black pepper. Heat the olive oil in a large cast iron skillet over medium-high heat. Place the beef tenderloin in the skillet and cook until they reach your desired degree of doneness; to cook to medium rare, it will take about 5 minutes per side. Transfer the beef to a serving platter and set aside.

Add the garlic and 2/3 of the parsley to the skillet and cook for 30 seconds, stirring regularly. Add the beef broth, butter and the brandy and cook over medium-high heat until the sauce is reduced to a glaze – this should take about 5 minutes. Pour the glaze over the beef tenderloin filets, sprinkle with the remaining 1/3 of the parsley and serve.

Flaxseed Pizza

Number of servings: 4

Ingredients:

1 ½ cups flax seed meal
2 tsp baking powder
3 tbsp olive oil
½ cup water
3 large eggs, beaten
1 tsp salt
a pinch of sugar

Preparation:

Start by preheating your oven to 425 F while you mix together the flax seed meal, baking powder, salt and sugar. Add the water, olive oil and eggs and mix together to combine, then set aside for 5 minutes to thicken.

Oil a baking pan or parchment paper and spread out the dough. Place in the oven and bake for 18 minutes. Remove pizza crust from the oven, allow to cool for a few minutes, top with the ingredients of your choice and then return to the oven for about 10 minutes or until the toppings are cooked through and the crust becomes slightly crisp. Remove from the oven, allow to cool for a few minutes, slice and serve.

Black Bean Tostadas

Number of servings: 2

Ingredients:

1 can (15 – 16 ounces) refried black beans
2 small Roma tomatoes, diced
1 small white or yellow onion, diced
2 tbsp chopped cilantro
½ an avocado, peeled, seeded and diced
1 cup shredded romaine or Bibb lettuce
2 ounces shredded cheese (your choice)
2 tortillas
Salsa and lime wedges, for serving

Preparation:

Start by preheating your oven to 350 F. Once the oven has reached 350 degrees, place the tortillas on a baking sheet and bake for 10 minutes or until crisp. While the tortillas are baking, heat the refried black beans.

Remove the tortillas from the oven once crisp, then spread with refried beans, shredded cheese, lettuce, diced onion, tomato and chopped cilantro. Serve with salsa and lime wedges.

Portabella Mushroom "Pizzas"

Number of servings: 4

Ingredients:

4 portabella mushroom caps, thoroughly washed
6 ounces mozzarella cheese, shredded
2 medium Roma tomatoes, roasted
4 fresh basil leaves
2 cloves garlic, crushed
1 tsp olive oil (use extra virgin olive oil)
Salt and black pepper, to taste

Preparation:

Preheat your oven to broiling temperature. Lightly oil a baking sheet, slice the tomatoes thinly and arrange on the baking sheet. Roast the tomatoes in the broiler for 3 -4 minutes, turning once. Remove the tomatoes from the oven, transfer to a plate and set aside. Lower the oven to 450 F while you prepare the other ingredients.

In a small bowl, mix together the olive oil and crushed garlic. Rub the garlic and oil mixture on all sides of the mushroom caps and place them, gill side up, on the baking sheet and sprinkle with a little salt and black pepper.

Top each mushroom cap with tomato slices, shredded mozzarella cheese and a basil leaf and place in the oven. Bake for 7 – 10 minutes, or until the cheese begins to brown.

Main Dishes

Baked Nutty Halibut

This is a delicious almond crusted baked halibut. Makes 4 servings.

What You'll Need:

4 halibut fillets

1 egg

1 lemon (cut into small wedges)

1 slice of rice bread

1/2 cup of almonds (slivered)

1/4 cup of milk

2 tablespoons of parsley (fresh chopped)

Salt and pepper

How to Make It:

Prep: Preheat the oven to 350 degrees Fahrenheit.

Toast the slice of rice bread; allow drying out, and then crumbling into fine breadcrumbs. In a bowl, add the egg and beat with a whisk, then stir in the 1/4 cup of milk.

Combine the breadcrumbs along with the 1/2 cup of almonds (slivered) and the 2 tablespoons of parsley (fresh chopped) in a separate bowl. Generously add dashes of salt and pepper to both sides of the halibut. Next, dip each seasoned halibut fillet in the milk and egg mixture, then roll in the nut mixture and place in a baking dish and bake for 5 to 10 minutes or until fish is done. Garnish with the lemon wedges.

Baked Parmesan Eggplant

This is a delicious main dish without meat, just eggplant, cheeses and a tasty crust.

What You'll Need:

2 slices of rice bread (brown)
1 eggplant (half inch slices)
1 cup of mozzarella cheese (shredded)
1 cup of tomatoes (Italian style canned, chopped)
1/2 cup of Parmesan cheese (grated)
1 tablespoon of avocado oil (extra virgin)
Salt and pepper

How to Make It:

Prep: Preheat the oven to 400 degrees Fahrenheit. Spray a baking sheet with cooking spray.

Toast the 2 slices of brown rice bread and create fine bread crumbs. Set the sliced eggplant on the prepared baking sheet. Shake a couple of dashes of salt and pepper over each slice. Bake the seasoned eggplants in the hot oven for 11 minutes. After baked, place the baked eggplants onto a platter.

Turn the oven heat down to 350 degrees Fahrenheit. Spray an 8x10 inch baking dish with cooking spray. Add the layers as follows 4 times: eggplant, 1/4 cup of the Italian tomatoes (chopped), 1/4 cup of the mozzarella cheese, and 1/8 cup of grated Parmesan cheese. Add the bread crumbs on top and then bake for about 15 minutes in the hot oven.

Baked Shrimp

This is a delicious baked shrimp made with coconut and seasoned with hot red pepper. Makes 8 servings.

What You'll Need:

2 pounds of shrimp (deveined, peeled)

1 cup of coconut (unsweetened, shredded)

1 cup of egg whites

8 tablespoons of coconut flour

1 tablespoon of agave nectar

1 tablespoon of lime juice

1/2 teaspoon of pepper (ground red)

Salt

How to Make It:

Prep: Preheat the oven to 425 degrees Fahrenheit. Spray a baking sheet with cooking spray.

Combine the 8 tablespoons of coconut flour, 1/2 teaspoon of pepper (ground red), and a couple of dashes of salt in a bowl. In a separate bowl, combine the 1 tablespoon of agave nectar and 1 tablespoon of lime juice with a whisk. Add the cup of egg whites and continue stirring with the whisk. Sprinkle the 1 cup of coconut (unsweetened, shredded) onto a platter. Run each of the 2 pounds of peeled, deveined shrimp through the flour mixture first, then dip in the egg mixture, and then roll in the shredded coconut. Place each prepared shrimp onto the greased baking sheet and bake in the hot oven for 15 minutes.

Bean Burrito

Prepare a delicious Mexican dish with this black bean burrito. Makes 6 servings.

What You'll Need:

3 brown rice tortillas (cut in half to make 6 semi-circles)

2 cans of black beans (16 oz.)

3 cups of romaine lettuce

1 1/2 cups of scallions (chopped)

3/4 cup of salsa

1/2 cup of Monterey Jack cheese

1/3 cup of cilantro (fresh chopped)

1 tablespoon of chilies (chopped, chipotle with adobo sauce)

1 1/2 teaspoons of cumin (ground)

How to Make It:

Combine the 2 cans of black beans (16 oz.), 1 tablespoon of chilies (chopped, chipotle with adobo sauce), and 1 1/2 teaspoons of cumin (ground) in a saucepan and turn to medium heat. After it simmers add the 1 1/2 cups of scallions (chopped) and the 1/3 cup of cilantro (fresh chopped) and cook for a couple of minutes. Lay the 6 semi-circle brown rice tortillas open and evenly divide the bean mixture onto the center of each tortilla piece. Divide the 3 cups of romaine lettuce and the 1/2 cup of Monterey Jack cheese in the same manner. Roll up into half burritos. Serve each burrito with 2 tablespoons of salsa.

Blackened Salmon

This is a delicious fish and rice dish. Makes 4 servings.

What You'll Need:

4 salmon fillets
4 lemon wedges
1 cup of brown rice (cooked)
1/3 cup of parsley (flat-leaf, fresh chopped)
1/4 cup of lemon juice
3 tablespoons of butter
2 tablespoons of paprika
1 teaspoon of thyme (dried)
1/2 teaspoon of cayenne pepper
1/2 teaspoon of garlic powder
Salt

How to Make It:

Prep: Preheat the oven to 400 degrees Fahrenheit.

Combine the 2 tablespoons of paprika, 1 teaspoon of thyme (dried), 1/2 teaspoon of cayenne pepper, 1/2 teaspoon of garlic powder, and a couple of dashes of salt in a cup. Add the 2 tablespoons of butter to a saucepan and turn to medium heat. Stir in the 1/4 cup of lemon juice. Put an oven-proof skillet on medium high heat. Take a salmon fillet, run it through the lemon butter, then roll it through the spices, and place in the hot skillet, cook for 2 minutes, flip, and cook for another 2. Repeat the process 3 more times with each of the salmon fillets. Put the fillets in the skillet and place in the hot oven for 8 minutes. Meanwhile add the final tablespoon of butter to the cooked rice (make sure the rice is hot) and toss in the 1/3 cup of parsley (flat-leaf, fresh chopped) and a few dashes of salt. Divide the rice over 4 plates, place a cooked salmon fillet over the rice and garnish with a lemon wedge.

Shrimp Stir Fry with Asparagus

This is a delicious stir fry with tomatoes, asparagus, and seasoned with cilantro. Makes 4 servings.

What You'll Need:

3/4 pound of asparagus (trimmed, cut to a little over an inch)
3/4 pound of shrimp (peeled, deveined, frozen)
1 cup of tomatoes (chopped)
3/4 cups of cilantro (fresh chopped)
1/2 cup of chicken stock
1 tablespoon of olive oil (extra virgin)
1 teaspoon of garlic (minced)
Spaghetti squash (cooked, enough for 4 servings)
Water

How to Make It:

Rinse the 3/4 pound of shrimp (peeled, deveined, frozen) by running cold water over it. Fill a six quart pan half way with water and turn to high heat to bring to a boil. Add the rinsed shrimp to the boiling water and cook for 3 minutes. Drain the water. Clean the pan and set it back on medium high heat. Add the 1 tablespoon of olive oil (extra virgin) and sauté the 3/4 pound of asparagus (trimmed, cut to a little over an inch) and the 1 teaspoon of garlic (minced) for a couple of minutes. Add the 1 cup of tomatoes (chopped), 3/4 cups of cilantro (fresh chopped), and the 1/2 cup of chicken stock and stir. When it boils, turn the heat to medium and add the shrimp to heat through for a couple of minutes. Serve over a bed of spaghetti squash.

Veggie Burger

This delicious burger does not have an ounce of meat in it; instead, it contains primarily black beans. Makes 4 servings.

What You'll Need:

1 can of black beans (16 oz.)
2 eggs
1 cup of onion (fine chopped)
1/4 cup of bell pepper (green, fine diced)
1/4 cup of flax seeds (ground)
1/2 tablespoon of chili powder
2 teaspoons of garlic powder
1 1/2 teaspoon of garlic (minced)
1 teaspoon of cumin (ground)
Salt and pepper

How to Make It:

Prep: Preheat the oven to 375 degrees Fahrenheit. Spray a baking sheet with cooking spray.

Add the can of black beans to a bowl and using a potato masher, mash into a paste. Mash in the 1 cup of onion (fine chopped), 1/4 cup of bell pepper (green, fine diced,

2 teaspoons of garlic powder, 1 1/2 teaspoon of garlic (minced), and dashes of salt and pepper. In a separate bowl crack the 2 eggs and beat with a whisk, and then combine with the 1/2 tablespoon of chili powder and 1 teaspoon of cumin (ground). Add the egg mixture into the mashed beans, mashing to combine well. Add the 1/4 cup of flax seeds (ground) and mashed until mixed. Make 4 burger patties and place them on the baking sheet and bake for 10 minutes, flip, and bake another 10 minutes.

Side Dishes

White Beans With Swiss Chard

Number of servings: 4

Ingredients:

1 can (15 – 16 ounces) white beans; either cannellini or great northern beans is fine

4 cups Swiss chard or rainbow chard, washed, patted dry and chopped

6 sundried tomatoes, chopped

½ cup vegetable broth

4 cloves garlic, sliced thinly

2 tbsp olive oil (use extra virgin olive oil)

Salt and black pepper, to taste

Preparation:

Bring 6 cups of lightly salted water to a boil in a large saucepan or stockpot. Add the Swiss chard and boil for 5 minutes until they turn bright green and take on a crisp-tender texture. Drain and set aside.

Put the saucepan back on the heat, add the vegetable broth cook over medium-high heat. Add the sliced garlic and the white beans and cook for another 1 -2 minutes to heat through the beans. Add the Swiss chard back to the pan and cook for another 2 minutes. Remove from heat, drizzle with olive oil, season to taste with salt and black pepper and serve using a slotted spoon to drain off excess moisture.

Zucchini and Sardine Salad

Number of servings: 2

Ingredients:

1 medium sized zucchini or yellow squash, sliced thinly

1 can sardines, drained

1 tbsp fresh dill, chopped (use more if you like – dried dill can be substituted if necessary)

Juice of 1 lemon

2 tbsp olive oil (use extra virgin olive oil)

Salt and black pepper, to taste

Preparation:

Mash the sardines with a fork and mix together in a bowl with the zucchini slices and dill. In a separate, smaller bowl mix together the olive oil, lemon juice and a little salt to make a dressing. Pour the dressing over the zucchini and sardine mixture, toss to coat, season to taste with salt and black pepper and serve. This recipe can also be prepared using anchovies in the place of sardines, if desired.

Moroccan-Spiced Roasted Vegetables

Number of servings: 4

Ingredients:

1 bunch asparagus, trimmed and cut into 1" pieces
1 medium sized parsnip, trimmed and cut into 1" pieces
1 large or 2 medium carrots, trimmed and cut into 1" pieces
1 large red or yellow onion, diced
1 leek, trimmed, cleaned thoroughly and sliced into 1" pieces
4 cloves garlic, halved
2 tbsp olive or coconut oil
3 tsp Ras el Hanout*
Salt, to taste

Preparation:

Preheat your oven to 425 F while you prepare the vegetables. Toss the chopped vegetables with the olive or coconut oil, a little salt and Ras el Hanout.

Line a cookie sheet or baking dish with parchment paper and arrange the vegetables in a single layer. Bake until vegetables are nicely browned, about 45 minutes; you may want to turn them once about halfway through.

* If you're unfamiliar with Ras el Hanout (literally, "top of the shop"), this is a Moroccan spice blend available at Middle Eastern groceries and some health food stores. If you can't find Ras el Hanout where you live, you can make a similar spice mix with cumin, coriander, cinnamon, clove, red and black pepper, nutmeg and turmeric. This recipe is also good with other spice blends such as Indian garam masala, Ethiopian berebere or if you're so inclined, even less exotic blends like Old Bay (although you'll want to omit any added salt if you're using a spice mix which contains salt).

Wild Rice Pilaf

Number of servings: 4

Ingredients:

½ cup wild rice, uncooked
½ cup brown rice, uncooked
2 ½ cups water or vegetable broth (omit salt if using broth)
1 ½ tbsp olive oil
1 tbsp fresh ginger, peeled and minced
½ cup dried apricots, sliced thin
¼ cup sunflower seeds (preferably raw)
½ tsp cinnamon
½ tsp cayenne pepper (use more or less to taste)
a pinch of salt, if not using vegetable broth

Preparation:

Bring water and salt to a boil in a large pot. While the water heats, rinse the wild rice and once the pot comes to a boil, add the wet rice and reduce the heat to medium. Cook, covered for 10 minutes, then rinse the brown rice and add it to the pot. Reduce the heat to a simmer and cover. Cook until the wild and brown rice are both done, about 40 minutes.

When the rice is cooked, heat the olive oil over low heat in a small pan along with the cayenne pepper, cinnamon and sliced apricots. Cook until aromatic, about 3 minutes, stirring occasionally. Stir in the apricot-spice mixture and the sunflower seeds. This dish can be served immediately while still warm, allowed to cool to room temperature or refrigerated and served cold.

Lima Bean Hummus

Number of servings: 4

Ingredients:

1 15 ounce can of lima beans, drained and rinsed
Juice of 2 lemons
2 cloves garlic, minced
1 tbsp fresh Italian parsley, minced
½ tsp cumin
1 tsp olive oil
Salt, to taste
A pinch of paprika

Preparation:

Place the drained lima beans, garlic, lemon juice, cumin, olive oil and a little salt in a food processor and process until it reaches the desired consistency. If you'd like your lima bean hummus to be a little thinner, then you can add a little extra lemon juice or a teaspoon of water at a time until you arrive at the consistency you like. Transfer to a bowl, stir in the minced parsley and refrigerate for 2 hours before serving, topped with a sprinkling of paprika.

Warm Goat Cheese Salad

Number of Servings: 2

Ingredients:

1 medium sized tomato, halved
2 ½ inch slices of goat cheese
2 tsp pesto
Arugula

Preparation:

Preheat your oven to 325 F. Slice the tomatoes in half and spread each with 1 tsp pesto and top with a slice of goat cheese. Place the tomato halves on top of a bed of arugula on oven-safe plates and bake for a few minutes to allow the goat cheese to soften and the arugula to wilt slightly. Serve warm.

Seaweed Salad

Number of servings: 8

Ingredients:

2 cups dried seaweed (hijiki or arame)
4 cups water
1 medium sized cucumber, diced (peeling and seeding are optional)
1 small carrot, shredded
3 green onions, sliced
½ cup fresh Italian parsley, chopped
Juice of 2 lemons
2 tbsp toasted sesame oil
1 ½ tbsp tamari or Bragg's liquid aminos

Preparation: Rinse the seaweed well and soak in 4 cups water until rehydrated. Drain well and mix together with the remaining ingredients and toss. Serve at once or refrigerate – this salad keeps well in the refrigerator for up to 4 days.

Sesame Cucumber "Noodles"

Number of servings: 4

Ingredients:

2 medium cucumbers
2 tsp sesame seeds, toasted
1 tbsp toasted sesame oil
1 tbsp tamari or Bragg's liquid aminos
Crushed red pepper, to taste

Preparation:

Peel the cucumbers and trim off the ends. The easiest way to proceed from here is to cut the cucumbers in half so that they're easier to handle and use a mandoline to slice the cucumbers thinly lengthwise to form flat noodle-like shapes – although this can also be done with a sharp knife and steady hands.

Slice the cucumbers, rotating as you cut until you reach the seeds. Place the cucumber "noodles" in a bowl and toss with the toasted sesame oil, half of the toasted sesame seeds and tamari. Refrigerate for at least 1 hour to chill and allow the flavors to blend. Serve cold, sprinkled with the remaining toasted sesame seeds and crushed red pepper.

Salad Greens with Yogurt Tahini Dressing

Number of servings: 6

Ingredients:

5 cups romaine or Bibb lettuce, chopped
1 cup arugula, radicchio or chicory (or a mixture of all three), chopped
½ cup cilantro, chopped
1 medium carrot, grated
2 medium tomatoes, halved and sliced

For the dressing:

1/4 cup low fat yogurt
1/3 cup orange juice
4 tbsp tahini
1 tsp sesame oil (toasted or untoasted, either is fine in this recipe)
A pinch of cayenne pepper
Black pepper, to taste

Preparation:

Wash, drain and chop the lettuce and cilantro and put into a large salad bowl. Grate the carrot and stir into the greens. In a smaller bowl, mix the yogurt, sesame oil, tahini, orange juice, cayenne and black pepper using a whisk to blend thoroughly. Drizzle the yogurt tahini dressing over the salad, toss to mix and serve.

Tomato, Red Bean and Mushroom Soup

Number of servings: 4

Ingredients:

3 medium tomatoes, diced
1 15 ounce can red beans, drained and rinsed
1 cup sliced crimini mushrooms
½ of a small white, yellow or red onion, minced
2 cloves garlic, minced
1 celery stalk, diced
1 tbsp fresh cilantro, chopped
a dash of cardamom
2 tsp oil (olive or coconut)
4 cups water
salt and black pepper, to taste
lemon wedges and chopped cilantro, for serving

Heat the oil in a Dutch oven or medium sized saucepan over medium-low heat. Once the oil is hot, add the garlic and onion and sauté until browned, about 5 minutes, stirring regularly. Add the diced celery, mushrooms and tomatoes and continue to cook, stirring occasionally, for another 5 minutes, or until the mushrooms have softened and release their water. Add the cardamom, red beans and water and bring to a boil. Reduce the heat and simmer the soup, covered for 20 minutes. Taste and season as needed with salt and black pepper. Ladle into bowls and serve hot with chopped cilantro and lemon wedges.

Mushrooms With Blue Cheese

Number of servings: 4

Ingredients: 1 12 ounce package mushrooms (crimini are best for this recipe), washed and sliced
1 cup coconut milk
3 tbsp blue cheese (any other cheese you prefer may be substituted)
2 cloves garlic, minced
2 tbsp coconut oil
Black pepper, to taste

In a small saucepan, sauté the sliced mushrooms and garlic in coconut oil over medium heat until the garlic is browned, about 4 minutes, stirring regularly to prevent burning.

Add the cheese and coconut milk and cook over medium-low heat, stirring frequently, until the mixture thickens. Serve hot with whole grain toast points or whole grain crackers.

Steamed Artichokes With Lemon Butter

Number of servings: 4

Ingredients:

4 artichokes, washed
1 stick butter
4 lemons
1 tbsp mustard seeds
1 tbsp coriander seeds
2 tsp salt
black pepper, to taste

Preparation:

Place 4 quarts of water in a large pot and bring to a boil over high heat. While the water is heating up, trim the stems of your artichokes, leaving about 2". Squeeze 2 of the lemons and add their juice to the boiling water along with their peels, salt and the mustard and coriander seeds.

Add your artichokes to the pot and cover them with a lid smaller than the pot or a plate to keep them submerged in the boiling water. Boil for 15 minutes and check for doneness; your artichokes will be done when you can insert a knife where the stem meets the bottom of the flower and remove it easily.

When the artichokes are almost done, melt the stick of butter in a small saucepan, then add the juice of the other 2 lemons and season to taste with salt and black pepper. Serve one artichoke to each diner, along with a small dish of the lemon butter and a bowl to place their discarded leaves.

Arugula and Grilled Chicken Salad

Number of servings: 4

Ingredients:

3 cups arugula, washed and drained of excess moisture
8 ounces grilled chicken, sliced thin
4 radishes, sliced thin
1 green onion, sliced into thin rounds
1 medium sized avocado, peeled, seeded and sliced

For the dressing:

2 tbsp extra virgin olive oil
1 tsp honey
Juice of 2 limes
A pinch of salt
Black pepper, to taste

In a small bowl, mix the olive oil, honey, lime juice, salt and black pepper with a whisk to mix well. Divide the arugula into 4 individual bowls and top with sliced green onion, radishes, grilled chicken and avocado. Serve with dressing on the side.

Green Beans With Gorgonzola Cheese and Walnuts

Number of servings: 4

Ingredients:

4 cups fresh green beans, trimmed
¼ cup walnuts, chopped
¼ cup vegetable or chicken broth
1 ounce gorgonzola cheese, crumbled
3 tsp walnut or extra virgin olive oil
Salt and black pepper, to taste

Preparation:

Add the green beans and broth to a large skillet and bring to a boil, then reduce to a simmer and steam the beans for 5 – 7 minutes, until they're slightly tender but still a little crisp. Remove the skillet from heat and transfer the green beans to a serving dish. Top with the crumbled gorgonzola cheese and chopped walnuts, sprinkle with salt and black pepper and serve.

Braised Leeks

Number of servings: 4

Ingredients:

8 leeks, trimmed and quartered lengthwise
¼ cup vegetable broth
1 tbsp olive oil
Juice and zest of ½ lemon
A pinch of salt
Black pepper, to taste

Preparation:

Preheat your oven to 425 F. Quarter the leeks and wash thoroughly under cold running water, then place in a baking pan covered in cold water and allow to soak for 15 minutes to loosen any remaining sand or dirt. Rinse the leeks again and set aside.

Coat a large baking dish with nonstick cooking spray, place the quartered leeks in the disk and drizzle with olive oil. Bake for 10 minutes, uncovered and turn over before baking for another 10 minutes. Pour the broth, lemon juice and zest over the leeks and bake for another 10 minutes, until they become tender. Season with a pinch of salt and black pepper and serve.

Sardine Pate

Ingredients:

1 can sardines in olive oil, drained
1 tbsp kalamata olives, chopped
2 sun dried tomatoes, chopped finely
¼ of a small red onion (1 – 2 tbsp), chopped finely
Black pepper, to taste

Preparation:

Drain the sardines and place them in a small bowl. Mash the sardines to a uniformly smooth consistency using a fork. Mix in the chopped sun dried tomatoes, chopped red onion and chopped olives and stir well to combine. Refrigerate for 1 -2 hours and serve cold with whole grain crackers.

Mashed Sweet Potatoes With Chipotle

Number of servings: 4

Ingredients:

4 medium sized sweet potatoes, washed and cut into ½"
slices
2 tbsp chipotle peppers in adobo sauce, chopped finely
3 tbsp milk
1 tbsp butter
Salt and black pepper, to taste

Preparation:

Boil the sweet potatoes until soft, about 15 minutes.
Drain and place the cooked sweet potato slices in a large
bowl and mash until smooth. Add the butter, chipotle
peppers in sauce and milk and stir until well combined.
Season to taste with salt and black pepper and serve.

Bean Salad

This quick and easy salad makes a great light lunch too.
Makes 4 servings.

What You'll Need:

1 can of chick peas (drained, rinsed)

3 cups of arugula (torn into pieces)

1/2 cup of lemon juice

1/2 cup of olive oil (extra virgin)

1/2 cup of tomatoes (chopped)

1/3 cup of onion (sliced)

1 tablespoon of lemon zest

1 tablespoon of salt

1 1/2 teaspoon of garlic (minced)

How to Make It:

Combine the 1/2 cup of lemon juice, 1/2 cup of olive oil
(extra virgin),
1 tablespoon of lemon zest, 1 tablespoon of salt, and 1
1/2 teaspoon of garlic (minced) in a bowl with a whisk.
Pour into a salad dressing bottle and set in the
refrigerator. In a large bowl combine the 1 can of chick
peas (drained, rinsed), 3 cups of arugula, 1/2 cup of
tomatoes (chopped), and 1/3 cup of onion (sliced) and

toss. Drizzle desired amount of dressing over each serving. Store unused dressing in the refrigerator.

Cauliflower Mushroom Nut Stuffing

This is an excellent side dish made with hazelnuts and crimini mushrooms. Makes 8 servings.

What You'll Need:

1 pound of mushrooms (crimini, diced)

1 cauliflower head (florets)

1 cup of celery (sliced)

1 cup of hazelnuts

1/2 cup of butter (divided)

1/2 cup of leeks (chopped)

1/3 cup of parsley (fresh chopped)

1/4 cup of lemon juice (divided)

1 tablespoon of thyme (fresh chopped)

1/2 tablespoon of sage (fresh, fine chopped)

1/3 tablespoon of lemon zest

1 teaspoon of garlic (minced)

Salt

How to Make It:

Prep: Preheat the oven to 350 degrees Fahrenheit. Spray a 13x9 inch baking dish with cooking spray.

Place a skillet on medium heat and add the 1/4 cup of

butter. Stir in the 1 pound of mushrooms (crimini, diced), 1 cup of celery (sliced), and 1/2 cup of leeks (chopped) and sauté for 5 minutes. Pour the sautéed mushrooms, celery, and leeks into the prepared 13x9 inch baking dish. Toss in the 1 cauliflower head (broken into florets). Melt the remaining 1/4 cup of butter and combine the 1 cup of hazelnuts, 1/8 cup of lemon juice, 1 tablespoon of thyme (fresh chopped), 1/2 tablespoon of sage (fresh, fine chopped), 1/3 tablespoon of lemon zest, 1 teaspoon of garlic (minced), and a couple of dashes of salt into a food processor or blender and pulse to break up the hazelnuts into a ground meal. Add the nut mixture over the mushrooms and vegetables and toss to mix. Bake in the hot oven for 40 minutes. Pull from oven and stir, then increase the temperature to 375 degrees Fahrenheit and bake for another 40 minutes. Stir every 20 minutes. Cool for a few minutes, then sprinkle the remaining 1/8 cup of lemon juice over the top prior to serving.

Cheesy Artichokes and Tomatoes

This is a savory side dish made with Swiss cheese, artichokes and tomatoes. Makes 4 servings.

What You'll Need:

3 tomatoes (sliced)

1 can of artichoke hearts (14 oz., sliced)

1 cup of Swiss cheese (shredded)

1/2 cup of basil (fresh chopped)

2 tablespoons of olive oil (extra virgin)

Salt and pepper

How to Make It:

Prep: Preheat the oven to 400 degrees Fahrenheit. Spray a 1.5 quart casserole dish with cooking spray. Layer the dish as follows: 3 tomatoes (sliced) and 1 can of artichoke hearts (14 oz., sliced). Next, add the 1/2 cup of basil (fresh chopped) and dashes of salt and pepper. Top with the cup of shredded Swiss cheese and finally pour the 2 tablespoons of extra virgin olive oil on top. Bake in the hot oven for 20 minutes, or until the top turns a nice golden brown. Cool for a few minutes before serving.

Grape Onion and Arugula Salad

This is a different twist using roasted red grapes to bring the salad to a new level of flavor. Makes 4 servings.

What You'll Need:

2 ounces of Parmesan cheese (sliced)

8 cups of arugula (torn to pieces)

2 cups of grapes (red, seedless)

3 onions (peeled, cut in half)

4 tablespoons of olive oil (extra virgin)

1 1/2 tablespoons of balsamic vinegar

1 teaspoon of Dijon mustard

1 teaspoon of thyme (fresh chopped)

Salt and pepper

How to Make It:

Prep: Preheat the oven to 375 degrees Fahrenheit. Line a baking sheet with parchment paper. Add the 2 cups of grapes (red, seedless) and the 3 onions (peeled, cut in half) to the baking sheet, keeping separate. Bake for 20 minutes, turning grapes 3 times. Remove the grapes to a bowl and continue to bake the onions for another 20 minutes. Remove the onions and place in a bowl to cool (not with the grapes). Add the cooled onions to a food processor or blender along with the 4 tablespoons of olive oil (extra virgin), 1 1/2 tablespoons of balsamic vinegar, 1 teaspoon of Dijon mustard, and dashes of salt and pepper. Process until smooth. Transfer to a bowl and stir in the 1 teaspoon of thyme (fresh chopped). Add the 8 cups of arugula (torn to pieces) and drizzle half of the dressing over the top and toss. Serve with the roasted red grapes and sliced Parmesan cheese. Drizzle more dressing if desired.

Mashed Baked Squash

This is a great substitute for mashed potatoes because squash is an excellent food to support thyroid health.

What You'll Need:

1 butternut squash
4 basil leaves (fresh)
1/2 cup of yogurt (lemon, room temperature)
1/2 cup of yogurt (vanilla, room temperature)

How to Make It:

Prep: Preheat the oven to 350 degrees Fahrenheit. Scrub the butternut squash and place it in a small baking dish and set the dish in the hot oven for 60 minutes. Set the baked squash on the counter top or cool stove to cool for about 10 minutes. Just like with a baked potato, cut the squash lengthwise in half. Remove the center seeds. Remove the outer skin. Combine the meat of the squash with the 1/2 cup of yogurt (lemon, room temperature) and 1/2 cup of yogurt (vanilla, room temperature) using a potato masher, until smooth consistency. Place in an oven-safe serving dish and reheat for about 10 minutes in the hot oven. Garnish each serving with a basil leaf.

Salmon Salad

Here is another great salad that makes a wonderful filling lunch. Makes 4 servings.

What You'll Need:

6 cups of arugula (torn to pieces)
2 cans of Salmon (drained)
4 radishes (sliced thin)
1 avocado (sliced)
1 tomato (chunked)
2 tablespoons of balsamic vinegar
2 tablespoons of olive oil (extra virgin)
1 teaspoon of honey
Salt and pepper

How to Make It:

Combine the 2 tablespoons of balsamic vinegar, 2 tablespoons of olive oil (extra virgin), 1 teaspoon of honey, and dashes of salt and pepper in a bowl with a whisk. Combine the 6 cups of arugula (torn to pieces), 2 cans of Salmon (drained), 4 radishes (sliced thin), 1 avocado (sliced), and 1 tomato (chunked) and toss. Drizzle the dressing over the top, toss to coat and serve immediately.

Sautéed Asparagus and Red Pepper

This is a delicious side dish of asparagus and the sweetness of red bell peppers. Makes 4 servings.

What You'll Need:

1 bell pepper (red, sliced)
4 cups of asparagus (trimmed)
1/4 cup of chicken stock

How to Make It:

Pour the 1/4 cup of chicken stock into a skillet and turn heat to medium high. When stock is heated, add the 4 cups of asparagus (trimmed) and the 1 bell pepper (red, sliced) on top. Cook for 6 minutes.

Shrimp Salad

Here is another tasty salad that makes for a great lunch as well. Makes 2 servings.

What You'll Need:

4 ounces of shrimp (deveined, peeled, cooked)
4 cups of arugula (torn into pieces)
2 tablespoons of orange juice
1 tablespoon of rice vinegar
1/2 teaspoon of orange peel (fine grate)
Pepper

How to Make It:

Combine the 2 tablespoons of orange juice, 1 tablespoon of rice vinegar, 1/2 teaspoon of orange peel (fine grate), and dashes of pepper in a small bowl with a whisk. Toss the 4 ounces of shrimp (deveined, peeled, cooked) and the 4 cups of arugula (torn into pieces) together. Drizzle the dressing over the top and toss to coat.

Breakfast

Asparagus and Sun-Dried Tomato Frittata

Number of servings: 4

Ingredients:

6 large or extra-large eggs
1 cup asparagus, blanched and cut into 1" pieces
¼ cup sun dried tomatoes, chopped finely
½ of a small red onion, diced
¼ cup milk
1 tbsp butter
2 tbsp parmesan or Romano cheese, grated
Black pepper, to taste

Preparation:

Preheat your oven to 325 F. Beat the eggs in a large bowl along with the milk, Romano or parmesan cheese and a little black pepper.

In a medium sized cast iron skillet, melt the butter over medium high heat and add the diced onion. Sautee the onion about 3 minutes until it turns translucent, stirring occasionally. Add the egg mixture and reduce the heat to low, tilting the pan to ensure that the eggs cover the entire bottom of the pan. As soon as the eggs start to set, stir in the asparagus and sun dried tomatoes.

Transfer the skillet to the oven and cook for another 2-3 minutes or until the center puffs up and the eggs are completely cooked around the edges. Remove the skillet from the oven and invert over a serving platter to remove. Slice the frittata and serve immediately.

Ricotta Soufflés With Blackberries

Number of servings: 6

Ingredients:

For the ricotta soufflés:

2 cups (16 ounces) ricotta cheese
6 large eggs
2 tbsp sugar or an equivalent amount of sugar substitute
Zest of 1 lemon

For the blackberry compote:

2 cups blackberries (fresh is preferable, but frozen is also OK if blackberries aren't in season when you make this recipe)
Juice of 2 lemons
A pinch of sugar or sugar substitute

Preparation:

Start by making the blackberry compote. Place the blackberries in a small pan with a pinch of sugar and the juice of 2 lemons. Stir and heat over medium-low heat, stirring occasionally until the blackberries soften.

Reduce the heat to low and keep warm.

While you're making the blackberry compote, preheat your oven to 375 F. Butter 6 muffin tins or ramekins (you can also use cooking spray, if desired). Mix together the eggs, sugar or sugar substitute and lemon zest in a bowl, using a whisk to combine. Add the ricotta cheese and continue whisking until a smooth mixture is formed. Pour into the muffin tins or ramekins and bake for 15 minutes.

Top the ricotta soufflés with blackberry compote and bake for another 15 minutes or until the soufflés are just set. Remove from the oven and either serve the soufflés right away while they're still warm or place them in the refrigerator for 1 – 2 hours and serve chilled.

Pumpkin-Coconut Pancakes

Number of servings:

Ingredients:

¼ cup cooked pumpkin (canned or homemade; butternut squash also works well)
¼ cup coconut milk
4 tbsp coconut meal
2 tbsp coconut oil
3 large eggs
1 tsp cinnamon
1 tsp nutmeg
½ tsp vanilla extract
¼ tsp baking soda
a pinch of sugar
a pinch of salt

Preparation:

Heat a nonstick skillet over medium heat. While the skillet heats, whisk together the coconut meal, salt, sugar, nutmeg, cinnamon and baking soda in a large bowl. In a smaller separate bowl, whisk together the eggs, vanilla extract, pumpkin and coconut milk.

Add the dry ingredient mixture to the egg mixture gradually, whisking to combine as you go. Add coconut oil to the skillet, tilting to coat the entire bottom of the pan. Spoon batter into the pan and shape pancakes with the spoon, since the batter will be thicker than traditional pancake batter.

Watch the pancakes carefully as they cook; they don't bubble like most pancakes, so you'll need to look at the edges to see how they're coming along. They should take 1 ½ to 2 minutes per side; when they're golden brown on the bottom, flip and cook the other side. Serve hot with butter and a drizzle of honey or real maple syrup.

Eggs Benedict With Salmon And Artichokes

Number of servings: 4

Ingredients:

8 large eggs
8 large artichoke bottoms
2 ounces smoked salmon
¼ cup Greek yogurt
2 tbsp cream cheese, softened
2 tbsp olive oil
2 tsp oregano (fresh or dried)
Juice and zest of ¼ of a lemon
Salt and black pepper, to taste

Preparation:

Preheat your oven to 425 F. Brush the artichoke bottoms on both sides with 1 tbsp olive oil and sprinkle with oregano. Once the oven reaches 425 F, place the artichokes on a baking sheet, top side facing down and make for 13 – 15 minutes or until the artichokes begin to brown.

While the artichokes are baking, mix together the Greek yogurt, cream cheese, lemon juice and a little water (about 1 tsp) in a bowl using a whisk until smooth and set aside. In a separate, larger bowl, beat the eggs and heat 1 tbsp olive oil in a large skillet over medium high heat. When the oil is hot, add the eggs and cook to your desired doneness.

When it's time to serve, divide the roasted artichoke bottoms between 4 plates and top each artichoke with smoked salmon, an egg and the yogurt – lemon sauce. Sprinkle with the remaining oregano, season to taste with salt and black pepper and serve.

Eggs Florentine Wraps

Number of servings: 2

Ingredients:

4 large or extra-large eggs
4 tbsp cheese (your choice), shredded or crumbled
1 cup raw baby spinach
2 tsp olive oil
A splash of milk (about 2 tsp)
1 large (burrito size) tortilla
Salt and black pepper, to taste

Preparation:

Crack the eggs into a medium sized mixing bowl and beat well with a splash of milk while you heat a skillet over medium heat. Add the olive oil to the skillet when the skillet is hot and tilt to coat the bottom thoroughly.

Add the spinach to the pan and cook until just wilted (about 1 minute), then pour in the eggs over the spinach and cook, stirring regularly until just set, about 2 minutes. Remove from heat, season with a little salt and black pepper and top with the cheese. Cover the skillet to help melt the cheese.

Toast the tortilla over the flame of a gas stove; if you have an electric stove, you can also warm your tortilla in a dry skillet over high heat (just a few seconds per side) or in a microwave. Fill the tortilla with the egg and spinach mixture, fold up burrito-style, slice in half and serve.

Mushroom And Cheddar Omelet

Number of servings: 2

Ingredients:

4 large eggs

¾ cup sliced mushrooms (crimini, button or any other mushrooms you prefer)

2 tbsp sharp cheddar cheese, grated

2 tbsp red onion, diced finely

1 tsp olive oil

A splash of milk (about 2 tsp)

A pinch of salt

Black pepper, to taste

Preparation:

Crack the eggs into a medium sized mixing bowl, add milk and beat well to combine while you heat the olive oil in a skillet over medium heat. Add the diced red onion and sauté for 1 minute, followed by the mushrooms. Cook for an additional 2 minutes, or until the mushrooms begin to soften, stirring occasionally. Pour the eggs over the mushrooms and cook until the omelet is set on the bottom. Distribute the grated cheese evenly over the top of the omelet, fold in half and continue cooking for another 1 – 2 minutes, or until the eggs have just set and the cheese is melted. Slice the omelet in half and serve.

Quinoa Breakfast Porridge

Number of servings: 2

Ingredients:

1 cup quinoa, uncooked
2 cups water
1 cup fresh or frozen, thawed blueberries
2 tbsp flax seeds
1 tsp sugar or an equivalent amount of sugar substitute
A pinch of salt

Preparation:

Start by rinsing the quinoa well in a sieve; quinoa must be rinsed before cooking to remove bitter tasting compounds found on the surface of the seed. Many commercially available brands of quinoa have already been rinsed to remove this coating, but if you buy your quinoa in bulk or you just want to be sure, go ahead and rinse it first.

Add the rinsed quinoa and 2 cups water to a small saucepan and bring to a boil, then reduce to a simmer and cook for about 15 minutes or until the quinoa is tender and the water is almost entirely absorbed. Stir in the blueberries, flax seeds, sugar and salt and cook for another 1 – 2 minutes. Remove from heat, stir and serve.

Asparagus Omelet

What a delicious way to start a day than with an omelet made with fresh asparagus. Makes 2 servings.

What You'll Need:

6 asparagus spears (cut into bit sized strips)
4 eggs
1/2 cup of water
1/4 cup of onion (diced)
2 teaspoons of olive oil
Salt and pepper

How to Make It:

Add the 1/2 cup of water to a skillet and turn to high to bring to a boil. Cook the 6 asparagus spears (cut into bit sized strips) for half a minute. Remove from water and place in a bowl of cold water to stop the cooking, drain the water. Add dashes of salt. Pour the 2 teaspoons of olive oil in the skillet and turn to medium heat. Spread the oil and sauté the 1/4 cup of onion (diced) for about 3 minutes. Put the onions on a plate. Turn the heat to medium low. Crack the 4 eggs and beat with a whisk. Add dashes of salt and pepper. Pour the eggs into the skillet and allow to cook into an omelet. When the bottom is cooked, carefully flip the eggs to cook the other side. Add the cooked asparagus and onions and fold the egg over omelet style. Remove omelet before it browns. Serve immediately.

Blueberry Muffins

If you have a sweet tooth you will love blueberry muffins for breakfast. Makes 1 dozen muffins.

What You'll Need:
6 eggs
1 cup of blueberries
1/2 cup of coconut flour
4 tablespoons of coconut oil
3 tablespoons of agave nectar
1 tablespoon of vanilla extract
1/2 teaspoon of baking soda
1/2 teaspoon of salt

How to Make It:

Prep: Preheat the oven to 350 degrees Fahrenheit.
Place 12 cupcake papers in a 12 cup muffin tin.

Combine the 1/2 cup of coconut flour, 1/2 teaspoon of
baking soda, and 1/2 teaspoon of salt in a bowl and set
aside. Crack the 6 eggs into a large bowl and beat with a
whisk. Combine the eggs with 4 tablespoons of coconut
oil, 3 tablespoons of agave nectar, and 1 tablespoon of
vanilla extract. Gradually add in the dry ingredients
mixing well. Fold in the 1 cup of blueberries and spoon
evenly into the dozen lined muffin tin. Bake until tops
turn a golden brown, about 23 minutes. Cool for 10
minutes on a wire rack.

Appetizer and Snack Recipes

Basic Guacamole

Guacamole is a favorite among those that enjoy spicier dishes. Makes 1 bowl.

What You'll Need:

2 avocados (chopped and mashed)
1 tomato (finely chopped)
1/4 cup of onion (finely chopped)
1/2 teaspoon of garlic (minced)
2 tablespoons of cilantro (fresh, fine chopped)
Dash of lemon juice
Dash of lime juice
Salt

How to Make It:

Combine the 2 avocados (chopped and mashed), 1 tomato (finely chopped), 1/4 cup of onion (finely chopped), 1/2 teaspoon of garlic (minced), 2 tablespoons of cilantro (fresh, fine chopped), Dash of lemon juice, Dash of lime juice, and a couple of dashes of salt in a bowl. Using a large fork or a potato masher, mash all the ingredients together. Store in the refrigerator but eat the same day it is made.

Fruit Nut Salad

This salad is great as a snack but can also make for a nice breakfast or lunch. Makes 8 servings.

What You'll Need:

4 cups of salad greens
2 pears chopped)
1 apple (sliced thin, cored)
1 cup of pecans (halved)
1 cup of feta cheese (crumbled)
1/2 cup of onion (sliced thin)
1 egg white
6 tablespoons of balsamic vinegar
2 tablespoons of honey
2 tablespoons of olive oil (extra virgin)
1 teaspoon of cinnamon (ground)
Salt and pepper

How to Make It:

Prep: Preheat the oven to 325 degrees Fahrenheit.   Add

the egg white to a bowl and beat with a whisk for a few seconds. Add the 2 tablespoons of honey and the teaspoon of ground cinnamon and mix well. Stir in the cup of halved pecans and toss to coat. Spread the coated pecans on a baking sheet and bake for 20 minutes. Remove sheet from the oven and let cool completely. Combine the
2 pears (chopped), 1 apple (sliced thin, cored), 1 cup of feta cheese (crumbled), and 1/2 cup of onion (sliced thin). Toss in the cooled pecans. Combine the 6 tablespoons of balsamic vinegar, 2 tablespoons of olive oil (extra virgin), and dashes of salt and pepper in a small bowl. Toss the fruit and nut mixture in with the 4 cups of salad greens. Drizzle the dressing over the top and toss. Serve immediately.

Granola

Granola makes a great snack or a quickie breakfast if you are on the run. Makes about 5 cups of granola.

What You'll Need:

2 cups of almonds
1 cup of macadamia nuts
1 cup of pumpkin seeds
1 cup of raisins
1 tablespoon of vanilla extract
1/2 teaspoon of cinnamon (ground)
Salt
Water

How to Make It:

Prep: The day before - Combine the 2 cups of almonds, 1 cup of macadamia nuts, and the 1 cup of pumpkin seeds in a bowl. Cover with water. In a smaller separate bowl, add the 1 cup of raisins and just barely cover with water. Soak both bowls overnight. The next morning preheat the oven to 250 degrees Fahrenheit. Either spray a baking sheet with cooking spray or line it with parchment paper. Next, pour the raisins and water into the food processor or blender and process until smooth.

Rinse the soaked nuts and add to the pureed raisins in the blender or food processor. Process until it is coarse chopped. Add the 1 tablespoon of vanilla extract, 1/2 teaspoon of cinnamon (ground), and a couple of dashes of salt and process for a few more seconds to combine, but not pulverize. Spread the mixture over the prepared baking sheet and bake in the hot oven for 45 minutes. Allow to cool completely before serving. Store in a zipper bag in the refrigerator.

Desserts

Flourless Chocolate Cake

Number of servings: 8

Ingredients:

12 ounces bittersweet chocolate

8 large eggs, separated

1/3 cup sugar or an equivalent amount of sugar substitute

1 ½ sticks of butter

3 tsp vanilla extract

¼ tsp cream of tartar

¼ tsp salt

Preparation:

Preheat your oven to 325 F. Oil a 9" spring form cake pan and lightly flour the pan (with coconut flour, if you have it on hand, otherwise any flour will do). Cover the bottom of the pan with a piece of parchment paper and set aside.

Melt the butter and bittersweet chocolate together in a double boiler over low heat until smooth. Remove from heat and allow to cool slightly.

Beat the egg whites in a mixing bowl until they become frothy. Add the cream of tartar and sugar or sugar substitute and continue to beat the mixture until stiff peaks form – think of making meringue. Don't overbeat the eggs; if you do, they'll curdle and you'll have to discard the mixture and start all over again.

Add the egg yolks and vanilla to the melted chocolate and butter mixture, using a whisk to combine thoroughly. Fold the egg white mixture into the chocolate gently until a light, fluffy mixture forms. Pour the batter into your prepared spring form cake pan.

Cover the bottom of the cake pan with aluminum foil and place on a baking dish filled with about ½" of water. Place the baking dish in the oven and bake for 65 – 70 minutes, or until a toothpick inserted in the center of the cake comes out clean.

Remove the cake from the oven and allow it to cool for an hour before removing from the pan. To remove the cake from the pan, use a knife; run it gently around the inside of the edge and invert carefully onto a plate.

Remove the parchment paper from the cake and invert again onto a serving plate. Refrigerate the cake for at least 6 hours and preferably overnight before serving; it's OK to eat the cake once it's cooled and removed from the pan, but it both look and taste best after it's had several hours or longer to set and chill in the refrigerator.

No Bake Pumpkin Bites

Number of servings: varies

Ingredients:

8 ounces dates, chopped (1 cup packed full)
1 cup rolled oats
1 cup toasted coconut
1 cup toasted pumpkin seeds
¼ cup cooked pumpkin (canned or homemade)
¼ cup honey
1 tbsp flax seeds
1 tsp powdered ginger
1 tsp cinnamon
½ tsp nutmeg
a pinch of salt

Preparation:

Add the pumpkin, honey, dates, flax seeds, spices and salt to a food processor and mix until smooth. Remove the mixture from the food processor and transfer to a large mixing bowl. Stir in the toasted pumpkin seeds, toasted coconut and rolled oats until combined. Place the bowl in the refrigerator, covered, for 1 hour.

After the mixture has chilled, use a spoon to portion out and shape the mixture into the size and shape you like (about 1" balls or rough cubes is good). Store refrigerated in a covered container; these no bake pumpkin bites will keep for 10 – 14 days.

Coconut Cheesecake Bars

Number of servings: varies

Ingredients:

1 cup cream cheese, softened at room temperature
1 cup coconut flour
1 stick of butter
4 large eggs
3 tbsp sugar or an equivalent amount of sugar substitute
2 tsp vanilla extract
1 tsp coconut oil

Preparation:

Preheat your oven to 350 F. Oil a large baking dish (11" x 7") with coconut oil and set aside. Beat the butter and cream cheese with an eggbeater or handheld electric mixer to incorporate air until a fluffy mixture is formed. Beat eggs into the mixture one at a time and mix well, followed by the sugar or sugar substitute, coconut flour and vanilla extract, beating each ingredient into the mixture.

Pour the batter into the prepared baking dish and bake for 30 minutes or until set. Allow the bars to cool to room temperature, refrigerate for at least 2 hours. Cut the coconut cheesecake bars into squares and serve chilled.

Coffee Custard

Number of servings: 4

Ingredients:

2 extra large eggs, beaten
1 ½ cups milk
2 tbsp sugar or an equivalent amount of sugar substitute
2 tsp espresso grounds
1 tsp vanilla extract
Cinnamon and lemon wedges, for serving

Preparation:

Add the beaten eggs, milk, sugar or sugar substitute, espresso grounds and vanilla extract to a medium sized mixing bowl and whisk together to combine. Divide the mixture among 4 ramekins or custard cups. Place the cups in a large skillet filled with enough water to reach up to ½" from the cups and bring to a boil over high heat before reducing to low and simmering, covered, for 10 minutes.

Remove the cups from the skillet and seal each with plastic wrap and refrigerate for 2 hours. Serve chilled, garnished with lemon wedges and cinnamon.

Coconut Rum Ice Cream

Number of servings: varies

Ingredients:

2 cups coconut milk

¾ cup sugar or an equivalent amount of sugar substitute

3 tbsp coconut oil

1 yolk from an extra large egg

1 tbsp vanilla extract

1 tbsp non alcoholic rum flavoring

A pinch of salt

Preparation:

Over low heat, whisk together the coconut milk, coconut oil, sugar or sugar substitute and salt until the sugar and salt are dissolved. Remove from heat and allow to cool to room temperature. Add the mixture to a blender with the vanilla extract, rum extract and egg yolk; blend until smooth.

If you have an ice cream maker, pour the mixture in and freeze according to the manufacturer's directions. If not, you can freeze the mixture overnight in a tightly covered glass bowl in your freezer. Serve your coconut ice cream on its own or with the (sensible) toppings of your choice.

Conclusion

As you have no doubt discovered while reading through (and hopefully preparing and enjoying) the recipes in this cookbook, there is an entire world of culinary options out there for people with hypothyroidism. As long as you stick to the basic rules – a healthy diet which is low in refined carbohydrates and sugars and includes plenty of high quality, lean proteins and fresh fruits and vegetables, you'll be able to get the nutrition you need to manage your condition; and you won't have to feel like you're missing out on anything at the dinner table.

These recipes follow the same basic formula of any healthy diet – which means that even if you're the only person in your household who suffers from hypothyroidism, the recipes in this book are also healthy choices for everyone else at your table. In fact, preparing these recipes for your family and getting them involved in a healthy diet can go a long way towards helping you to keep your hypothyroidism under control and getting your energy back. Having the support of your loved ones is invaluable when you're trying to recover from or manage any disorder and hypothyroidism is no different. With a little help from your family and friends, you'll find that it's easy to eat right, have the energy to get regular exercise and generally manage your hypothyroidism effectively so that you can live your life again; and that definitely includes having a good time preparing and enjoying meals!